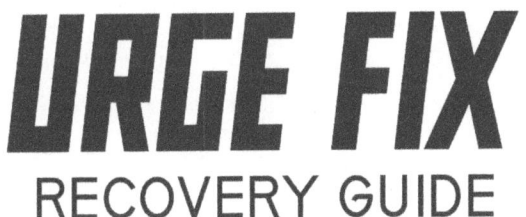

URGE FIX
RECOVERY GUIDE

URGE FIX
RECOVERY GUIDE

Cyntrell T. Crawford,
MD, MPH

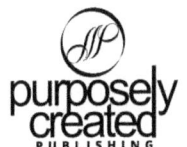

URGE FIX RECOVERY GUIDE
Published by Purposely Created Publishing Group™
Copyright © 2018 Cyntrell Crawford

All rights reserved.

No part of this book may be reproduced, distributed or transmitted in any form by any means, graphic, electronic, or mechanical, including photocopy, recording, taping, or by any information storage or retrieval system, without permission in writing from the publisher, except in the case of reprints in the context of reviews, quotes, or references.

Limit of Liability / Disclaimer of Warranty: While the publisher and author have used their best efforts in preparing this book, they make no representations or warranties with the respect to the accuracy or completeness of the contents of this book and specifically disclaim any implied warranties of fitness for a particular purpose. No warranty may be created or extended by sales representatives or written sales materials. The advice and strategies contained herein may not be suitable for your situation. You should consult with a doctor where appropriate. Neither the publisher nor author shall be liable for any loss or damages including but not limited to special, incidental, consequential or other damages.

Printed in the United States of America
ISBN: 978-1-948400-78-7

Special discounts are available on bulk quantity purchases by book clubs, associations and special interest groups.
For details email: sales@publishyourgift.com
or call (888) 949-6228.

For information logon to:
www.PublishYourGift.com

This book is dedicated to:

My family,

Vonda,

And those in recovery who inspire me every day.

Table of Contents

Foreword 1

CHAPTER 1
Addiction Is a Disease 5

CHAPTER 2
Acceptance 9

CHAPTER 3
Pros and Cons 17

CHAPTER 4
Prepare to Change 21

The Urge Fix Action Plan 23

CHAPTER 5
Support System 29

CHAPTER 6
Recovery and Preventing Relapse 35

Thank You 39

About the Author 41

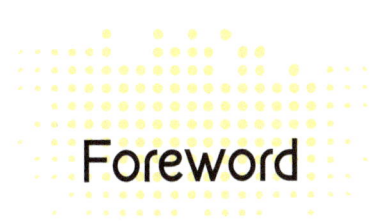

Foreword

Anthropologists have documented the earliest known substance use by human beings at around 35,000 years ago. Substances have been used and abused by every culture, population, and religion on the face of the earth. Substance use and abuse transcend history, culture, and family values.

Recently, mankind has produced a number of chemicals designed to help society and individuals. During World War II, the Japanese used Ma Huang (a root with amphetamine-like properties) to help workers stay awake during wartime production. When the supply ran short, they were able to synthesis methamphetamine (a drug which can both help a child with ADHD and destroy the life of a loved one or an entire community).

In the 1960's, man synthesized a drug to help pregnant women with morning sickness. Thalidomide worked miracles on nausea but caused an entire generation of children with severe birth defects.

Morphine and opium have been around forever. There are stories about the opium houses in the 1800's and about using opium in everything from tonic water to teething medicines for babies. It is very effective for pain relief in the short-term and highly addictive in the long-term.

Substance abuse, drug addiction, is a very complex problem. No one wakes up one morning and decides to become addicted to oxycodone, crystal meth, or heroin. But, people do! Not because of a moral failure or a lack of understanding the dangers, but for simple reasons which can often go very wrong.

In this book, Cyntrell Crawford, a psychiatrist, provides a clear, focused, and understandable plan for beginning the battle against your addiction. She makes no promises that your fight will be easy or brief. There is no judgment to be found in the following pages. Instead, Dr. Crawford provides a clear roadmap for beginning your journey to sobriety and a drug-free life.

Read each chapter quickly, then go back and read each one again––slowly. Let the wisdom sink in. Carry this book with you and open it to any page when you are having trouble with thoughts of relapse. It takes up very little room in your pocket and it can help your journey toward a better life!

Excelsior,
Harvey Norris, LCSW

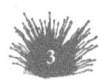

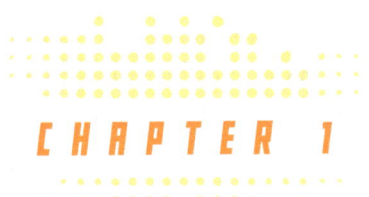

CHAPTER 1
Addiction Is a Disease

There is so much debate regarding addiction being a moral failure versus a disease. My thought about that debate is, "Who the hell cares? People are dying daily from addiction and we need to help them recover." My understanding of drug and alcohol addiction is that it is a progressive disease with the following hallmark indicators: developing tolerance to drugs, intense cravings, and withdrawal symptoms. The signs of addiction can be grouped into three categories: emotional, behavioral, and physical.

My clients show several emotional signs such as: being easily irritable with frequent anger outbursts, over-sensitivity to topics related to drug and alcohol usage, poor ability to deal with daily stressors, and the inability to experience pleasure from activities usually found satisfying. They also frequently use defense mechanisms such as: rationalizing (by making excuses for drug and alcohol usage), minimizing behaviors, and blaming others (explained later in this chapter).

The behavioral signs shown are: difficulty fulfilling their commitments and obligations, problems with the legal system (examples: DUI and public intoxication charges), disrupted sleep patterns, and poor relationships with their spouse, family members, and friends.

Some of the physical signs shown by my clients are: dilated pupils, red eyes, disheveled appearance, weight loss or appearance of malnutrition, and generally poor hygiene.

Some undercover, but very noticeable, signs in patients with drug and alcohol problems are:

1. **"Is that water?"** Vodka, or other clear alcoholic beverages, can become the drink of choice for alcoholics who want to hide their drinks in water bottles or other containers that would go unnoticed at work, home, or a doctor's or counselor's office.

2. **"Doc, I'm so anxious and I have multiple panic attacks daily."** Anxiety and panic attacks are frequent complaints from my patients with substance use. Anxiety and panic attacks are common side effects of many drugs, marijuana, alcohol, and even stimulants. Due to changes in

brain chemistry, these temporary symptoms can become long-lasting results of substance use.

3. **Blaming others.** Do you tend to blame others for your behaviors? It is normal for a person dealing with substance use to tell lies or minimize their involvement in a situation surrounding substance use. It is either blatant lies to cover up use, possible memory lapse, or difficulty admitting to yourself your role in the problem. What I really hear? "I'm not to blame, Doc. It was my mother, it was my friend, it was my dog, Charlie."

4. **Reasons.** Overtime, patients with drug and alcohol addiction usually develop tolerance which requires increased frequency and quantity of their drug of choice. Prescription drug users will reveal themselves by requesting prescription refills sooner. They will call the office to complain that they lost their prescription or they will say, "I had a fire in my apartment and my prescription was near the stove." "My prescription flew out of the window while driving home from the appointment." "The pharmacy did not give me the correct number of pills. I only got 75 and my prescription was written for 90." Those are just

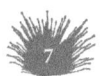

some of the reasons I have heard many times in my office.

> **Do you do any of these things? If you do, you might have a problem with drugs or alcohol.**

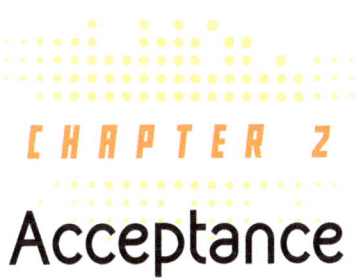

CHAPTER 2
Acceptance

Acceptance is key! But, it is often the hardest reality to face with drug and alcohol addiction. I have found that many of my clients often struggle with this first step as it goes against everything they want to do. I often hear, "They say I drink too much, but I just have a few beers every now and then." Further inquiry into what a few beers is leads to a discussion about more than the recommended daily consumption of alcohol. Also, they admit that quantity has led to many problems such as: not showing up for work, black outs, jail time, etc. These problems do not just stem from alcohol use. My clients with drug problems have the same reality. But, even with severe consequences, they don't see the problem as a problem. That is often due to not accepting their reality.

WHAT IS ACCEPTANCE?

Simply put, acceptance is agreeing to what is, not what you want it to be; and, recognizing the problem whether positive or negative, comfortable or uncomfortable, without changing or protesting. Furthermore, I tell my clients, "It isn't about what others say about you. You have to be even more selfish than your family or friends say you are now. This step is necessary for your survival." So, I have a discussion with them about self-acceptance, which is affirming within yourself that you have a weakness for drugs or alcohol. You must embrace all of yourself, good and bad, to move forward in your recovery and more importantly your life.

WHY IS ACCEPTANCE SO IMPORTANT?

Without acceptance of your drug and alcohol problems, how will you move forward? My simple answer to that question is, "You won't." Acceptance is one of the most important tools in recovering from drug and alcohol addiction. There are three common statements I've heard made by my clients suffering from drug and alcohol use: 1.) "I can't change." 2.) "Life sucks." 3.) "It isn't that big of a problem." Let's address these realities one by one.

1.) 'I CAN'T CHANGE.'

Changing your addiction and your life. Stages of change.

Change is a difficult but necessary process for recovery; it is not an instantaneous event. Instead, it often has to be done in small steps. Each small step is progress toward a bigger goal. So, even if you stumble during the process, your mistakes can become lessons.

Most addiction research studies discuss a model of change which involves five stages: pre-contemplation, contemplation, preparation, action, and maintenance. Each stage has strategies necessary for making a change. In the pre-contemplation stage, a person is usually not aware that a change is necessary. But, if they are aware, it's likely that they have had previous failed attempts at changing. In this stage, you must become aware of the problem and develop a goal for change. In the contemplation stage, there is some awareness, but the individual is usually noncommittal about making an effort to change. The preparation stage occurs when an individual starts making plans to change by researching the tools necessary for the change. The action ("money") stage is when an individual puts their research into action. In the maintenance stage, you have had consistent results toward your desired goal. This five stages model is usually presented in a circular format allowing for regression or relapse (as change is hard and movement through stages is not linear).

Some indications that a change will be successful are motivation for the change; setting a small, specific, real-

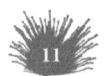

istic, tangible goal; avoiding your triggers; changing your environment; and, getting positive individuals to help you toward your goals.

Change is difficult; but, it is obtainable with the right tools, commitment, and persistence toward your recovery. For those who suffer from drug or alcohol addiction, change begins by stating, "I have a disease or illness that affects my ability to respond to alcohol or drug consumption in a manner conducive to appropriate daily living."

Although it is difficult, you can change. Accepting that there is a problem with your drug or alcohol use is vital to your success in recovery.

2.) "LIFE SUCKS."

Life sucking is not unique to you.

I have heard many reasons for drug and alcohol use. Some of those reasons are childhood trauma, rape, divorce, not having the desired career, homelessness, mental illness, boredom, and peer pressure. This is a simplified list that obviously cannot include every reason, and it might not include your reason. But, it is quite clear that life can be difficult at times. And honestly, no one makes it out alive.

As humans, we desire to avoid pain and experience pleasure. Individuals who suffer from addictions usually run from harsh realities and attempt to find comfort and pleasure while intoxicated. But, there is no way to run from suffering, pain, or loss. So, once you're no longer intoxicated, you must deal with your harsh reality. Then, the cycle continues as you repeatedly become intoxicated to avoid the pain. It is a catch-22 as most addictive behaviors add more pain to your life by affecting you, your family, and your friends. In plain terms, "Drugs take you to hell disguised as Heaven."

To live a life of recovery, you must face the harsh realities and learn to cope with suffering, pain, and loss by taking small, forward steps.

3.) "IT ISN'T THAT BIG OF A PROBLEM."

"Denial is more than a river in Africa" is a slogan often heard in recovery environments. Denial is a very common problem for clients who come to me with addictive behaviors. It maintains the addiction. Denial is the opposite of acceptance. It is refusing to accept what is and avoidance of the problem because it is uncomfortable and very unpleasant.

Denial is often the most difficult part of helping a person deal with their addiction because it is so engrained in their addictive behaviors. Denial helps them explain to themselves their use and justify continued use. Let's discuss forms of denial some of you struggling with addictive behaviors may relate to:

1. Rationalizing occurs when you make an excuse for doing what you want when you want. For instance: "I deserve this, I work hard every day." "I bought a new car. It's blue and I'm going to celebrate by drinking a blue can of liquor." "I'm going to die at the end anyway, why can't I smoke this cigarette?"

2. Blaming is diverting attention to another situation to avoid taking responsibility. For instance: "If you had a life like mine you would use also." "I was molested as a child and I used to stop the feelings."

3. Minimizing is discounting the severity of your addiction. For instance: "At least I'm not doing heroin." "Marijuana is legal in Colorado." "I'm not as bad as my father. He was a drunk."

4. Anger is used to push away those who voice concerns about your use. For instance: "I'm an adult, I don't need your advice!" "You drink also, why are you telling me to stop?"

5. Self-delusions are often used by people suffering from addiction to convince themselves that they don't have a problem at all. For instance: "I don't have to use, I can stop. I just don't feel like doing it now."

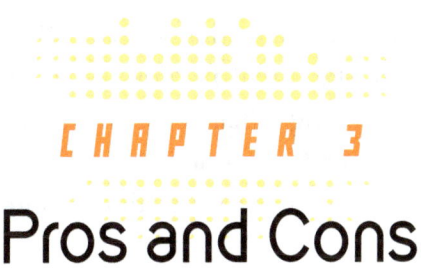

CHAPTER 3
Pros and Cons

Let's get down to it. Although I would love to say that there are no pros to drug and alcohol use, there must be some or there would be no need for this book. So, what are they? Simply put, euphoria and excitement.

Most individuals who deal with drug and alcohol addictive behaviors spend the majority of their time seeking and obtaining their next fix. They get their fix and bam… no more worries. No more problems with money, family, or fear. They are constantly chasing happiness, excitement, and their next escape.

A common complaint from my clients is, "I'm bored." That usually means, "I'm missing excitement." I am often confused by this complaint and recommend that they just go do something. Go to a movie, walk in a park, or read a book. Do anything, but don't use. With drug and alcohol use, the sensation of pleasure provides a sense of excitement, even if the person is not doing anything except sitting around and getting wasted with their friends. But, I do understand that in those times they feel as if they can do anything. Their senses are in overdrive, the world seems better, there is no pain, and jokes seem funnier. But, they are also prone to doing more dangerous things.

Most people who use drugs and alcohol have a fake confidence, prompting more dangerous and careless activities. Those feelings often lead to legal issues from driving while intoxicated (because they felt they could handle doing so), fighting strangers (because they feel stronger), or risky sexual behaviors (for fun or to help pay for more drugs and alcohol) leading to STDs, incarcerations, and unwanted pregnancy.

The BIGGEST con is the fake superhuman feelings. Those feelings are not real or long-lasting as you must continue to use drugs and alcohol to maintain them.

Can you think of some pros for stopping and cons for continuing your addictive behaviors? Here is some space for you to reflect. Let me help you start this exercise.

Examples:

Improving my relationships with family and friends.

No more hangovers, blackouts, or difficulty remembering my activities.

No more problems with the law (i.e., driving while intoxicated or public intoxication).

Keeping my job or continuing school.

	Pros	Cons

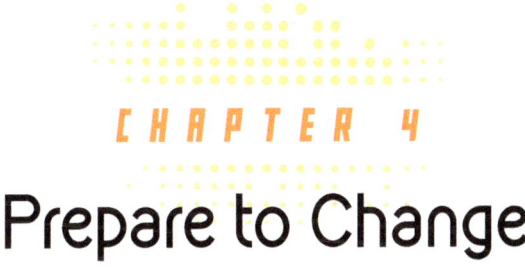

CHAPTER 4
Prepare to Change

Are you ready to change? This is a very tough decision. At times, you may have concerns about your ability to change (if you even want to). These mixed feelings are very common for anyone making big changes in their life. You will likely go back and forth with your decision until you are truly ready.

"No! I'm not quite ready. I'm definitely on the fence." Okay! Start by keeping track of your use. How often are you using and how much? At times, reexamine the pros of discontinuing your addiction and the reasons why changing will give you positive results in life. Evaluate what is stopping you from moving forward with your change. If necessary, seek professional help from family, friends, or your healthcare provider.

"Yes! I'm ready to change." If you are ready to change, it is helpful to develop a written plan to keep

track of your goals, why you are doing this, and how you plan to make it happen.

Here are questions to help you achieve your goals:

1. How will you keep track of your recovery? Example: write out a plan.

2. What are your goals? Example: I will stop using… because…

3. What will you do besides using drugs and alcohol? Example: I will attend an AA/NA meeting or I will watch a funny movie.

4. What has caused you to drink or use drugs?

5. What are your triggers? Example: stress, recent loss, new job.

6. How will you avoid people, places, and things that cause you to have the urge to use? Example: I will change my phone number. I will delete my dealer's number.

7. How will you keep yourself focused? Tip: Practice saying NO! It is a full sentence.

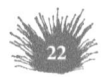

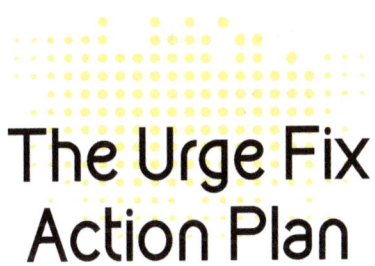

The Urge Fix Action Plan

WHAT IS THE URGE FIX ACTION PLAN?

The Urge Fix Action Plan is a guide to assist you in living a life of recovery.

WHY DOES IT WORK?

It works because it is easy to use and only for you. It will improve your communication with yourself, your family members, and your mental health care providers.

Use the space provided to write out your Urge Fix Action Plan.

WHAT ARE SOME THINGS THAT CAN HELP YOU BECOME BETTER DAILY?

Some strategies used by many seem basic and are often forgotten or overlooked. Here is a list to help you get started:

- Eating three healthy meals and two snacks
- Drinking plenty of water (approximately eight glasses)
- Maintaining your personal hygiene (grooming and taking a shower or bath)
- Exercising. Example: simply walking 30 minutes per day or every other day
- Writing in a journal
- Going to support group meetings
- Going to a movie

THE URGE FIX ACTION PLAN: HOW DO I LOOK WHEN I'M FEELING WELL?

It is often difficult to remember what your life was like when you were in good health, not struggling with your addiction or bad habit.

Use this space to recall how you were when you were feeling well. You can also use this space to picture how you would like to feel or live. Here is a list of words to help you get started.

I feel well when I am:

- ✅ responsible
- ✅ energetic
- ✅ smiling
- ✅ content
- ✅ present

I feel well when I am:

_____

_____

_____

_____

_____

THE URGE FIX ACTION PLAN: GOALS

You can use this space to write down your goals for your recovery. It can be as simple as: "I would like to get a job and go to work on time daily, go to school to learn a new skill, enjoy my family, and get into a relationship."

I will stop using… because…

___

My goals for my recovery:

___

Go back to the list of strategies we wrote earlier (i.e., eating healthy meals, going to support group meetings). These are the strategies you will use to do something besides drugs and alcohol.

The things I will put into action each day to support my recovery are:

_____

_____

_____

_____

_____

THE URGE FIX ACTION PLAN: TRIGGERS

Identifying a trigger is not easy. Triggers are external or internal circumstances that can cause stress, anxiety, a feeling of disappointment, or negative thinking. There are many kinds of triggers and they are normal occurrences. But, if you do not recognize them and learn to deal with them appropriately, they can lead you down a dangerous path and harm your recovery efforts. Some examples of common triggers include:

- ✅ exposure to the substance itself
- ✅ contact with people, places, and situations you associate with using (such as: your drinking or drugging buddies, parties, new situations, weekends)

- ✅ Some emotions such as: frustration, tiredness, stress, even happiness or a successful event can be a trigger

List your triggers:

_____

_____

_____

Below, make a strategy to overcome your triggers.

I will…

- ✅ remove myself from the situation
- ✅ go to a support group
- ✅ make a phone call to my support person and talk about my present situation
- ✅ pray or meditate

I will…

_____

_____

_____

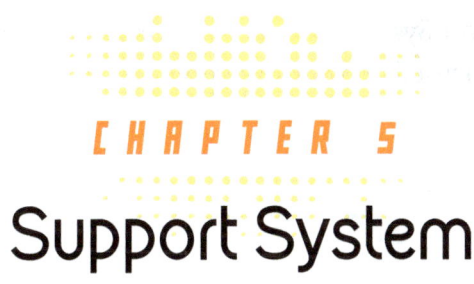

CHAPTER 5
Support System

HOW TO DEVELOP A SUPPORT SYSTEM

What do you need? Besides having a recovery plan, it is very important to build a support system. The support system should consist of friends and family who you can call on for support, encouragement, reality checks, or anything you may need during your recovery. These friends and family members should preferably be clean, sober, and not lead you down the wrong path in your recovery. No one from your life while you were drinking or drugging will do. These individuals need to know your goals and your plan for recovery. They have to be willing to take the journey with you.

Support System: who are the people you can call to get you focused on your recovery?

_____

_____

_____

_____

_____

Discussing your goals with family or friends. Family members can be an important component of your recovery. Some people will have family members who are actively involved in their recovery; others will not have that option. If your family members are involved, you should be very happy and appreciate the emotional support of having them by your side at this very important junction in your life. Please share your goals with your family members. They must know where you are in the process. Ask them to attend a meeting or two with you if you have decided to use a twelve-step program or therapy.

What do you need from your support system? While in recovery, never be afraid to ask for help with your situation. Asking for help is a sign of strength and growth.

Once you have developed your support system, make sure you have their contact information. Have frequent interaction with your family or friends by attending recovery meetings and having clean, sober fun (i.e., dinners). Make sure that your family or friends are aware of your goals which can simply be, "I don't want to drug or drink anymore." They need to fully support your recovery.

Before I forget, you should not have any guilt about removing people from your life who have a negative impact on your recovery. Addiction is a life or death situation. You do not need anyone in your life that would lead you back to drugs or alcohol. Those people no longer have a place in your life. Make sure you are surrounding yourself with people who will have a positive impact on your recovery.

Addiction can often be a very lonely process due to separating yourself from family members or friends because of your use. Recovery is and should be the complete opposite. To progress in your recovery, you must have a positive support system. This can be found in a twelve-step program that gives recovering addicts a safe place to talk about their addiction and recovery with other group members, and allows them to possibly find a sponsor (someone who provides additional support and accountability). The twelve-step program can be an extension of your family and friends or in place of them if you don't have a support system.

Others who should be added to your support system list are professional mental health practitioners. These are psychologists, licensed clinical social workers, professional counselors, and other licensed professionals who may help with substance use through counseling. They will help you work through your addiction by addressing:

Stress management techniques- It is very important to learn how to deal with stress in appropriate ways without substance use during your recovery. Develop proper coping skills to help reduce your chances of relapse. Some examples of coping skills are: calling someone on your support list and having a conversation, reading a book, taking a walk, praying, helping someone else, cleaning your house, watching a movie.

Coping Skills: list activities or skills you enjoy that can get your mind off drugs or alcohol.

_____

_____

_____

History of trauma- Unaddressed trauma can be a burden for many recovering addicts and can lead to relapse. A mental health professional can help you deal with your history of trauma.

Shame- A therapist can help you deal with your shame, guilt, or regrets from your active addiction. Discussion of these topics in a safe, non-judgmental environment can help you move forward with your life and possibly develop plans to mend your past.

Underlying mental health diagnosis- Many addicts, and those in recovery, often have other underlying issues such as: depression, anxiety, and bipolar disorder. A medical health professional can help counsel you or refer you to a psychiatrist.

It is very important to realize that the choice to use or not to use is up to you. While you are working hard to maintain your new, clean life, the people you allow in are a major part of your recovery plan. So, learn to recruit a support system which consists of emotionally supportive and positive people. They are in your life to help you help yourself.

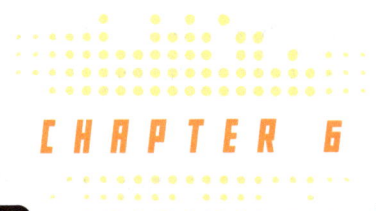

CHAPTER 6
Recovery and Preventing Relapse

Recovery is an active journey. In recovery, you have accepted your addiction, you are moving toward changing your behaviors, you are building a new life without your addictive behavior, and you are reducing your risk of relapse. You are also managing your recovery by working your recovery plan, engaging your support system, and possibly using self-help programs or a mental health professional. Now, you must learn to continue your recovery by active self-improvement. You must learn different things about yourself and your addiction, recovery, and how to prevent relapse.

Your number one priority in your new life is sobriety. It is important to stay away from the triggers you listed previously and to learn to manage your cravings. Don't worry, cravings tend to decrease in frequency and intensity as you stay away from drugs, alcohol, food, or cigarettes. Continue to use your support system for encouragement and to help you keep your mind focused on your recovery.

How do you prevent yourself from relapsing? Relapse is the reoccurrence of any disease that has been in remission or recovery. It is definitely a danger to your new life. You must always be aware of your thinking and feelings because signs of relapse are often very subtle, and before you know it, you are using again. Some of the feelings that make you vulnerable to relapse are usually described by the simple (but not all inclusive) acronym H.A.L.T.: Hungry, Angry, Lonely, or Tired. To reduce your chances of relapse and better your life, you will need to use your coping skills to get you through your daily activities. Also, check your thinking. Don't allow thoughts like, "I need a drink" or "I could use that cigarette" to creep into your mind as they could lead to relapse. Make sure your thoughts are focused on avoiding your addictive behaviors.

Keeping yourself on track or motivated is another priority in your recovery. Often during the early stages of recovery, a person has a high level of motivation to stay sober. But, as time goes on, this can decrease for many reasons. Relapse is a possibility when you let your motivation decrease. So, be sure to keep your recovery plan active. Continue with self-help programs, get new hobbies, or learn something new to keep your mind fresh. You can also help another person who is trying to recover. Reward yourself and celebrate your recovery as often as possible to remind yourself how far you have come.

Recovery is a life-long journey. It can be great at times and difficult at others. Just remember to maintain your recovery plan, build your support system, and seek help when necessary.

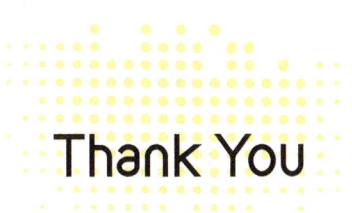
Thank You

Thank you for purchasing and reading this book. This is my first book and I would love your feedback. Don't be afraid, I don't bite and I can take it. My primary goal in my career and life is to grow daily. I hope you can utilize this information in your life and recovery. Spread the word and help me to assist as many people as possible!

I'm super busy either seeing a patient in one of my offices or doing an online, print, or media feature. And soon I'll be on the lecture circuit educating doctors, mental health professionals, or people like you about trends in addiction and recovery. Let's stay connected, so I can keep you updated on my activities and recovery tools.

WEBSITE:
https://www.DrCyntrell.com

FACEBOOK:
https://www.facebook.com/DrCyntrellPsych

TWITTER:
@DrCyntrellPsych

YOUTUBE:
DrCyntrellPsych

INSTAGRAM:
@DrCyntrellPsych

PINTEREST:
https://www.pinterest.com/DrCyntrellPsych

LINKEDIN:
https://www.linkedin.com/in/DrCyntrellPsych

GOOGLE+:
https://www.google.com/+DrCyntrellPsych

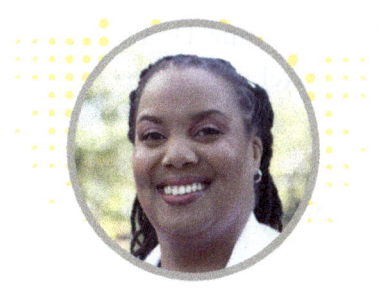

About the Author

Cyntrell T. Crawford, MD, is an adult psychiatrist, speaker, author, consultant, and media personality who is on a mission to provide life solutions for addiction and mental health. As the founder and chief medical advisor of DrCyntrell.com, she provides techniques to help individuals take control of their life through recovery. Dr. Cyntrell also shares mental health and addiction expertise via her web series.

Dr. Cyntrell earned her doctor of medicine from the Tulane University School of Medicine. She completed her internship and residency at the University of Texas Health Sciences Center at the Houston Department of Psychiatry and Behavioral Sciences. In addition, she holds a master of public health in health systems management. In her spare time, Dr. Cyntrell loves to read, try new things, and travel.

> **TO CONNECT, VISIT HER WEBSITE AT**
> **www.DrCyntrell.com**

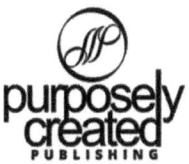

CREATING DISTINCTIVE BOOKS WITH INTENTIONAL RESULTS

We're a collaborative group of creative masterminds with a mission to produce high-quality books to position you for monumental success in the marketplace.

Our professional team of writers, editors, designers, and marketing strategists work closely together to ensure that every detail of your book is a clear representation of the message in your writing.

Want to know more?
Write to us at info@publishyourgift.com
or call (888) 949-6228

Discover great books, exclusive offers, and more at
www.PublishYourGift.com

Connect with us on social media

@publishyourgift

www.ingramcontent.com/pod-product-compliance
Lightning Source LLC
Chambersburg PA
CBHW070036040426
42333CB00040B/1697